HIGHPOINTERS LOGBOOK

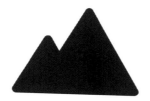

A Guided Journal to Record Climbing each State Summit in the United States

BY COLORFEST JOURNALS

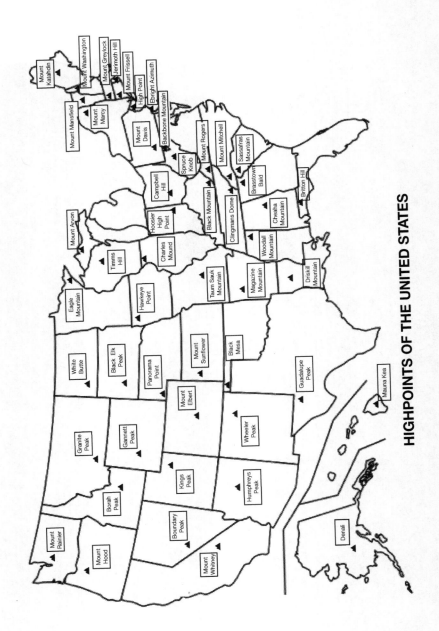

HIGHPOINTS OF THE UNITED STATES

Contents

State Highpoints Index
Mark your completed climbs to the summits

Alphabetical State Highpoints
Record your individual highpoint experiences

Address Book
For all the great Highpointers you meet along the way

HIGHPOINTS CLIMBED

Date

ALABAMA	Cheaha Mountain		
ALASKA	Denali		
ARIZONA	Humphreys Peak		
AKANSAS	Magazine Mountain		
CALIFORNIA	Mount Whitney		
COLORADO	Mount Elbert		
CONNECTICUT	Mount Frissell (south slope)		
DELAWARE	Ebright Azimuth		
FLORIDA	Britton Hill		
GEORGIA	Brasstown Bald		
HAWAII	Mauna Kea		
IDAHO	Borah Peak		
ILLINOIS	Charles Mound		
INDIANA	Hoosier High Point		
IOWA	Hawkeye Point		
KANSAS	Mount Sunflower		
KENTUCKY	Black Mountain		
LOUISIANA	Driskill Mountain		
MAINE	Mount Katahdin		
MARYLAND	Backbone Mountain		
MASSACHUSETTS	Mount Greylock		
MICHIGAN	Mount Arvon		
MINNESOTA	Eagle Mountain		
MISSISSIPPI	Woodall Mountain		
MISSOURI	Taum Sauk Mountain		

HIGHPOINTS CLIMBED

Date

MONTANA	Granite Peak		
NEBRASKA	Panorama Point		
NEVADA	Boundary Peak		
NEW HAMPSHIRE	Mount Washington		
NEW JERSEY	High Point		
NEW MEXICO	Wheeler Peak		
NEW YORK	Mount Marcy		
NORTH CAROLINA	Mount Mitchell		
NORTH DAKOTA	White Butte		
OHIO	Campbell Hill		
OKLAHOMA	Black Mesa		
OREGON	Mount Hood		
PENNSYLVANIA	Mount Davis		
RHODE ISLAND	Jerimoth Hill		
SOUTH CAROLINA	Sassafras Mountain		
SOUTH DAKOTA	Black Elk Peak		
TENNESSEE	Clingmans Dome		
TEXAS	Guadalupe Peak		
UTAH	Kings Peak		
VERMONT	Mount Mansfield		
VIRGINIA	Mount Rogers		
WASHINGTON	Mount Rainier		
WEST VIRGINIA	Spruce Knob		
WISCONSIN	Timms Hill		
WYOMING	Gannett Peak		

ALABAMA

CHEAHA MOUNTAIN - 2,407 ft   Date _____

WEATHER _____   TEMP _____

ROUTE _____

Easy   Moderate   Difficult   Strenuous

DISTANCE _____ ELEVATION GAIN _____

NOTES _____

_____

_____

_____

_____

_____

WHO WAS THERE

_____

_____

_____

_____

_____

THE EXPERIENCE

_____

_____

_____

_____

_____

_____

_____

_____

_____

_____

_____

☆ ☆ ☆ ☆ ☆

ALASKA

DENALI - 20,320 ft   Date_____

WEATHER _____ TEMP _____

ROUTE _____

Easy   Moderate   Difficult   Strenuous

DISTANCE _____ ELEVATION GAIN _____

NOTES _____

_____

_____

_____

_____

_____

_____

WHO WAS THERE

_____

_____

_____

_____

_____

_____

THE EXPERIENCE

☆ ☆ ☆ ☆ ☆

ARIZONA

HUMPHREYS PEAK - 12,633 ft   Date

WEATHER _____ TEMP _____

ROUTE _____

Easy   Moderate   Difficult   Strenuous

DISTANCE _____ ELEVATION GAIN _____

NOTES _____

WHO WAS THERE

THE EXPERIENCE

_____

_____

_____

_____

_____

_____

_____

_____

_____

_____

_____

☆ ☆ ☆ ☆ ☆

ARKANSAS

MAGAZINE MOUNTAIN-2,753 ft Date

WEATHER _____ TEMP _____

ROUTE _____

Easy   Moderate   Difficult   Strenuous

DISTANCE _____ ELEVATION GAIN _____

NOTES _____

_____

_____

_____

_____

_____

WHO WAS THERE

_____

_____

_____

_____

_____

_____

THE EXPERIENCE

☆ ☆ ☆ ☆ ☆

CALIFORNIA

MOUNT WHITNEY - 14,494 ft   Date

WEATHER _____ TEMP _____

ROUTE _____

Easy   Moderate   Difficult   Strenuous

DISTANCE _____ ELEVATION GAIN _____

NOTES _____

_____

_____

_____

_____

_____

WHO WAS THERE

_____

_____

_____

_____

_____

THE EXPERIENCE

☆ ☆ ☆ ☆ ☆

COLORAD0

MOUNT ELBERT - 14,433 ft   Date _____

WEATHER _____ TEMP _____

ROUTE _____

Easy   Moderate   Difficult   Strenuous

DISTANCE _____ ELEVATION GAIN _____

NOTES _____

_____

_____

_____

_____

_____

WHO WAS THERE

_____

_____

_____

_____

_____

THE EXPERIENCE

☆ ☆ ☆ ☆ ☆

CONNECTICUT

MOUNT FRISSELL - 2,380 ft   Date

WEATHER _____ TEMP _____

ROUTE _____

_____

Easy   Moderate   Difficult   Strenuous

DISTANCE ———————— ELEVATION GAIN ————

NOTES _____

_____

_____

_____

_____

_____

WHO WAS THERE

THE EXPERIENCE

⟡ ⟡ ⟡ ⟡ ⟡

DELAWARE

EBRIGHT AZIMUTH - 448 ft   Date

WEATHER _____ TEMP _____

ROUTE _____

Easy   Moderate   Difficult   Strenuous

DISTANCE _____ ELEVATION GAIN _____

NOTES _____

_____

_____

_____

_____

_____

WHO WAS THERE

_____

_____

_____

_____

_____

THE EXPERIENCE

☆ ☆ ☆ ☆ ☆

FLORIDA

BRITTON HILL - 345 ft   Date _____

WEATHER _____ TEMP _____

ROUTE _____

_____

Easy   Moderate   Difficult   Strenuous

DISTANCE _____ ELEVATION GAIN _____

NOTES _____

_____

_____

_____

_____

_____

WHO WAS THERE

_____

_____

_____

_____

_____

_____

THE EXPERIENCE

☆ ☆ ☆ ☆ ☆

GEORGIA

BRASSTOWN BALD - 4,784 ft   Date

WEATHER _____ TEMP _____

ROUTE _____

Easy   Moderate   Difficult   Strenuous

DISTANCE _____ ELEVATION GAIN _____

NOTES _____

_____

_____

_____

_____

_____

WHO WAS THERE

THE EXPERIENCE

☆ ☆ ☆ ☆ ☆

HAWAII

MAUNA KEA - 13,796 ft   Date

WEATHER _____ TEMP _____

ROUTE _____

Easy   Moderate   Difficult   Strenuous

DISTANCE _____ ELEVATION GAIN _____

NOTES _____

_____

_____

_____

_____

_____

WHO WAS THERE

THE EXPERIENCE

☆ ☆ ☆ ☆ ☆

IDAHO

BORAH PEAK - 12,662 ft   Date

WEATHER _____ TEMP _____

ROUTE _____

_____

Easy   Moderate   Difficult   Strenuous

DISTANCE _____ ELEVATION GAIN _____

NOTES _____

_____

_____

_____

_____

_____

WHO WAS THERE

_____

_____

_____

_____

_____

_____

THE EXPERIENCE

☆ ☆ ☆ ☆ ☆

ILLINOIS

CHARLES MOUND - 1,235 ft   Date

WEATHER _____ TEMP _____

ROUTE _____

_____

Easy   Moderate   Difficult   Strenuous

DISTANCE —————— ELEVATION GAIN ——————

NOTES _____

_____

_____

_____

_____

_____

WHO WAS THERE

_____

_____

_____

_____

_____

_____

THE EXPERIENCE

☆ ☆ ☆ ☆ ☆

INDIANA

HOOSIER HIGH POINT-1,257 ft Date _____

WEATHER _____ TEMP _____

ROUTE _____

_____

Easy   Moderate   Difficult   Strenuous

DISTANCE _____ ELEVATION GAIN _____

NOTES _____

_____

_____

_____

_____

_____

WHO WAS WITH YOU

_____

_____

_____

_____

_____

_____

THE EXPERIENCE

☆ ☆ ☆ ☆ ☆

IOWA

HAWKEYE POINT - 1,670 ft   Date _____

WEATHER _____ TEMP _____

ROUTE _____

Easy   Moderate   Difficult   Strenuous

DISTANCE _____ ELEVATION GAIN _____

NOTES _____

_____

_____

_____

_____

_____

WHO WAS THERE

_____

_____

_____

_____

_____

_____

THE EXPERIENCE

☆ ☆ ☆ ☆ ☆

KANSAS

MOUNT SUNFLOWER - 4,039 ft   Date _____

WEATHER _____ TEMP _____

ROUTE _____

_____

Easy   Moderate   Difficult   Strenuous

DISTANCE _____ ELEVATION GAIN _____

NOTES _____

_____

_____

_____

_____

_____

WHO WAS THERE

_____

_____

_____

_____

_____

_____

THE EXPERIENCE

☆ ☆ ☆ ☆ ☆

KENTUCKY

BLACK MOUNTAIN - 4,145 ft   Date_____

WEATHER _____ TEMP _____

ROUTE _____

Easy   Moderate   Difficult   Strenuous

DISTANCE _____ ELEVATION GAIN _____

NOTES _____

_____

_____

_____

_____

_____

WHO WAS THERE

_____

_____

_____

_____

_____

_____

THE EXPERIENCE

☆ ☆ ☆ ☆ ☆

LOUISIANA

DRISKILL MOUNTAIN - 535 ft Date _____

WEATHER _____ TEMP _____

ROUTE _____

Easy   Moderate   Difficult   Strenuous

DISTANCE _____ ELEVATION GAIN _____

NOTES _____

_____

_____

_____

_____

_____

WHO WAS THERE

_____

_____

_____

_____

_____

_____

THE EXPERIENCE

☆ ☆ ☆ ☆ ☆

MAINE

MOUNT KATAHDIN - 5,268 ft   Date _____

WEATHER _____ TEMP _____

ROUTE _____

Easy   Moderate   Difficult   Strenuous

DISTANCE _____ ELEVATION GAIN _____

NOTES _____

_____

_____

_____

_____

_____

WHO WAS THERE

_____

_____

_____

_____

_____

_____

THE EXPERIENCE

☆ ☆ ☆ ☆ ☆

MARYLAND

BACKBONE MOUNTAIN-3,360 ft Date

WEATHER _____ TEMP _____

ROUTE _____

Easy   Moderate   Difficult   Strenuous

DISTANCE _____ ELEVATION GAIN _____

NOTES _____

_____

_____

_____

_____

_____

WHO WAS THERE

_____

_____

_____

_____

_____

_____

THE EXPERIENCE

☆ ☆ ☆ ☆ ☆

MASSACHUSETTS

MOUNT GREYLOCK - 3,491 ft   Date

WEATHER _____ TEMP _____

ROUTE _____

Easy   Moderate   Difficult   Strenuous

DISTANCE _____ ELEVATION GAIN _____

NOTES _____

_____

_____

_____

_____

_____

WHO WAS THERE

THE EXPERIENCE

☆ ☆ ☆ ☆ ☆

MICHIGAN

MOUNT ARVON - 1,979 ft   Date _____

WEATHER _____ TEMP _____

ROUTE _____

_____

Easy   Moderate   Difficult   Strenuous

DISTANCE _____ ELEVATION GAIN _____

NOTES _____

_____

_____

_____

_____

_____

WHO WAS THERE

_____

_____

_____

_____

_____

THE EXPERIENCE

☆ ☆ ☆ ☆ ☆

MINNESOTA

EAGLE MOUNTAIN - 2,301 ft   Date_____

WEATHER _____ TEMP _____

ROUTE _____

_____

Easy   Moderate   Difficult   Strenuous

DISTANCE _____ ELEVATION GAIN _____

NOTES _____

_____

_____

_____

_____

_____

WHO WAS THERE

_____

_____

_____

_____

_____

THE EXPERIENCE

☆ ☆ ☆ ☆ ☆

MISSISSIPPI

WOODALL MOUNTAIN - 806 ft   Date _____

WEATHER _____ TEMP _____

ROUTE _____
_____

Easy   Moderate   Difficult   Strenuous

DISTANCE _____ ELEVATION GAIN _____

NOTES _____
_____
_____
_____
_____
_____

WHO WAS THERE

_____
_____
_____
_____
_____
_____

THE EXPERIENCE

☆ ☆ ☆ ☆ ☆

MISSOURI

TAUM SAUK MOUNTAIN-1,772 ft Date _____

WEATHER _____ TEMP _____

ROUTE _____

_____

Easy   Moderate   Difficult   Strenuous

DISTANCE ————————— ELEVATION GAIN —————

NOTES _____

_____

_____

_____

_____

_____

WHO WAS THERE

_____

_____

_____

_____

_____

_____

THE EXPERIENCE

☆ ☆ ☆ ☆ ☆

MONTANA

GRANITE PEAK - 12,799 ft   Date _____

WEATHER _____ TEMP _____

ROUTE _____

_____

Easy   Moderate   Difficult   Strenuous

DISTANCE _____ ELEVATION GAIN _____

NOTES _____

_____

_____

_____

_____

_____

WHO WAS THERE

_____

_____

_____

_____

_____

_____

THE EXPERIENCE

_____

_____

_____

_____

_____

_____

_____

_____

_____

_____

_____

☆ ☆ ☆ ☆ ☆

NEBRASKA

PANORAMA POINT - 5,424 ft   Date

WEATHER _____ TEMP _____

ROUTE _____

Easy   Moderate   Difficult   Strenuous

DISTANCE _____ ELEVATION GAIN _____

NOTES _____

_____

_____

_____

_____

_____

WHO WAS THERE

_____

_____

_____

_____

_____

_____

THE EXPERIENCE

☆ ☆ ☆ ☆ ☆

NEVADA

BOUNDARY PEAK - 13,140 ft   Date _____

WEATHER _____ TEMP _____

ROUTE _____

_____

Easy   Moderate   Difficult   Strenuous

DISTANCE _____ ELEVATION GAIN _____

NOTES _____

_____

_____

_____

_____

_____

WHO WAS THERE

_____

_____

_____

_____

_____

THE EXPERIENCE

☆ ☆ ☆ ☆ ☆

NEW HAMPSHIRE

MOUNT WASHINGTON - 6,288 ft Date _____

WEATHER _____ TEMP _____

ROUTE _____

_____

Easy   Moderate   Difficult   Strenuous

DISTANCE _____ ELEVATION GAIN _____

NOTES _____

_____

_____

_____

_____

_____

WHO WAS THERE

_____

_____

_____

_____

_____

_____

THE EXPERIENCE

☆ ☆ ☆ ☆ ☆

NEW JERSEY

HIGH POINT - 1,803 ft

Date _____

WEATHER _____ TEMP _____

ROUTE _____

_____

Easy   Moderate   Difficult   Strenuous

DISTANCE _____ ELEVATION GAIN _____

NOTES _____

_____

_____

_____

_____

_____

WHO WAS THERE

_____

_____

_____

_____

_____

_____

THE EXPERIENCE

_____
_____
_____
_____
_____
_____
_____
_____
_____
_____
_____

☆ ☆ ☆ ☆ ☆

NEW MEXICO

WHEELER PEAK - 13,161 ft   Date_____

WEATHER _____ TEMP _____

ROUTE _____

_____

.   Easy   Moderate   Difficult   Strenuous

DISTANCE _____ ELEVATION GAIN _____

NOTES _____

_____

_____

_____

_____

_____

_____

WHO WAS THERE

_____

_____

_____

_____

_____

_____

THE EXPERIENCE

☆ ☆ ☆ ☆ ☆

NEW YORK

MOUNT MARCY - 5,343 ft   Date_____

WEATHER _____ TEMP _____

ROUTE _____

Easy   Moderate   Difficult   Strenuous

DISTANCE _____ ELEVATION GAIN _____

NOTES _____

_____

_____

_____

_____

_____

WHO WAS THERE

_____

_____

_____

_____

_____

_____

THE EXPERIENCE

☆ ☆ ☆ ☆ ☆

NORTH CAROLINA

MOUNT MITCHELL - 6,684 ft   Date_____

WEATHER _____ TEMP _____
ROUTE _____

Easy   Moderate   Difficult   Strenuous

DISTANCE _____ ELEVATION GAIN _____

NOTES _____

_____

_____

_____

_____

_____

WHO WAS THERE

_____

_____

_____

_____

_____

_____

THE EXPERIENCE

☆ ☆ ☆ ☆ ☆

NORTH DAKOTA

WHITE BUTTE - 3,506 ft   Date

WEATHER _____ TEMP _____

ROUTE _____

_____

Easy   Moderate   Difficult   Strenuous

DISTANCE _____ ELEVATION GAIN _____

NOTES _____

_____

_____

_____

_____

_____

WHO WAS THERE

_____

_____

_____

_____

_____

_____

THE EXPERIENCE

☆ ☆ ☆ ☆ ☆

OHIO

CAMPBELL HILL - 1,550 ft   Date_____

WEATHER _____ TEMP _____

ROUTE _____

_____

Easy   Moderate   Difficult   Strenuous

DISTANCE _____ ELEVATION GAIN _____

NOTES _____

_____

_____

_____

_____

_____

WHO WAS THERE

_____

_____

_____

_____

_____

_____

THE EXPERIENCE

☆ ☆ ☆ ☆ ☆

OKLAHOMA

BLACK MESA - 4,973 ft   Date _____

WEATHER _____ TEMP _____

ROUTE _____

_____

Easy   Moderate   Difficult   Strenuous

DISTANCE _____ ELEVATION GAIN _____

NOTES _____

_____

_____

_____

_____

_____

WHO WAS THERE

_____

_____

_____

_____

_____

_____

THE EXPERIENCE

☆ ☆ ☆ ☆ ☆

OREGON

MOUNT HOOD - 11,239 ft   Date_____

WEATHER _____ TEMP _____

ROUTE _____

_____

Easy   Moderate   Difficult   Strenuous

DISTANCE _____ ELEVATION GAIN _____

NOTES _____

_____

_____

_____

_____

_____

WHO WAS THERE

_____

_____

_____

_____

_____

_____

THE EXPERIENCE

☆ ☆ ☆ ☆ ☆

PENNSYLVANIA

MOUNT DAVIS - 3,213 ft   Date

WEATHER _____ TEMP _____

ROUTE _____

_____

Easy   Moderate   Difficult   Strenuous

DISTANCE _____ ELEVATION GAIN _____

NOTES _____

_____

_____

_____

_____

_____

WHO WAS THERE

THE EXPERIENCE

☆ ☆ ☆ ☆ ☆

RHODE ISLAND

JERIMOTH HILL - 812 ft   Date _____

WEATHER _____ TEMP _____

ROUTE _____

_____

Easy   Moderate   Difficult   Strenuous

DISTANCE _____ ELEVATION GAIN _____

NOTES _____

_____

_____

_____

_____

_____

WHO WAS THERE

_____

_____

_____

_____

_____

_____

THE EXPERIENCE

☆ ☆ ☆ ☆ ☆

SOUTH CAROLINA

SASSAFRAS MOUNTAIN-3,560 ft Date _____

WEATHER _____ TEMP _____

ROUTE _____

_____

Easy   Moderate   Difficult   Strenuous

DISTANCE _____ ELEVATION GAIN _____

NOTES _____

_____

_____

_____

_____

_____

WHO WAS THERE

_____

_____

_____

_____

_____

_____

THE EXPERIENCE

☆ ☆ ☆ ☆ ☆

SOUTH DAKOTA

BLACK ELK PEAK - 7,242 ft   Date_____

WEATHER _____ TEMP _____

ROUTE _____

_____

Easy   Moderate   Difficult   Strenuous

DISTANCE _____ ELEVATION GAIN _____

NOTES _____

_____

_____

_____

_____

_____

WHO WAS THERE

_____

_____

_____

_____

_____

_____

THE EXPERIENCE

☆ ☆ ☆ ☆ ☆

TENNESSEE

CLINGMANS DOME - 6,643 ft   Date_____

WEATHER _____ TEMP _____

ROUTE _____

_____

Easy   Moderate   Difficult   Strenuous

DISTANCE _____ ELEVATION GAIN _____

NOTES _____

_____

_____

_____

_____

_____

WHO WAS THERE

_____

_____

_____

_____

_____

_____

THE EXPERIENCE

☆ ☆ ☆ ☆ ☆

TEXAS

GUADALUPE PEAK - 8,749 ft   Date_____

WEATHER _____ TEMP _____

ROUTE _____

_____

Easy   Moderate   Difficult   Strenuous

DISTANCE ──────── ELEVATION GAIN ────────

NOTES _____

_____

_____

_____

_____

_____

WHO WAS THERE

_____

_____

_____

_____

_____

THE EXPERIENCE

☆ ☆ ☆ ☆ ☆

UTAH

KINGS PEAK - 13,528 ft   Date

WEATHER _____ TEMP _____

ROUTE _____

Easy   Moderate   Difficult   Strenuous

DISTANCE _____ ELEVATION GAIN _____

NOTES _____

_____

_____

_____

_____

_____

WHO WAS THERE

_____

_____

_____

_____

_____

_____

THE EXPERIENCE

VERMONT

MOUNT MANSFIELD - 4,393 ft   Date_____

WEATHER _____ TEMP _____

ROUTE _____

Easy   Moderate   Difficult   Strenuous

DISTANCE _____ ELEVATION GAIN _____

NOTES _____

_____

_____

_____

_____

_____

WHO WAS THERE

_____

_____

_____

_____

_____

THE EXPERIENCE

☆ ☆ ☆ ☆ ☆

VIRGINIA

MOUNT ROGERS - 5,729 ft   Date_____

WEATHER _____ TEMP _____

ROUTE _____

_____

Easy   Moderate   Difficult   Strenuous

DISTANCE _____ ELEVATION GAIN _____

NOTES _____

_____

_____

_____

_____

_____

WHO WAS THERE

_____

_____

_____

_____

_____

_____

THE EXPERIENCE

☆ ☆ ☆ ☆ ☆

WASHINGTON

MOUNT RAINIER - 14,411 ft   Date_____

WEATHER _____ TEMP _____

ROUTE _____

_____

Easy   Moderate   Difficult   Strenuous

DISTANCE _____ ELEVATION GAIN _____

NOTES _____

_____

_____

_____

_____

_____

WHO WAS THERE

THE EXPERIENCE

☆ ☆ ☆ ☆ ☆

WEST VIRGINIA

SPRUCE KNOB - 4,863 ft   Date_____

WEATHER _____ TEMP _____

ROUTE _____

Easy   Moderate   Difficult   Strenuous

DISTANCE _____ ELEVATION GAIN _____

NOTES _____

_____

_____

_____

_____

_____

WHO WAS THERE

_____

_____

_____

_____

_____

THE EXPERIENCE

☆ ☆ ☆ ☆ ☆

WISCONSIN

TIMMS HILL - 1,951 ft   Date_____

WEATHER _____ TEMP _____

ROUTE _____

Easy   Moderate   Difficult   Strenuous

DISTANCE _____ ELEVATION GAIN _____

NOTES _____

_____

_____

_____

_____

_____

WHO WAS THERE

_____

_____

_____

_____

_____

_____

THE EXPERIENCE

_____

_____

_____

_____

_____

_____

_____

_____

_____

_____

☆ ☆ ☆ ☆ ☆

WYOMING

GANNETT PEAK - 13,804 ft   Date _____

WEATHER _____ TEMP _____

ROUTE _____

Easy   Moderate   Difficult   Strenuous

DISTANCE _____ ELEVATION GAIN _____

NOTES _____

_____

_____

_____

_____

_____

WHO WAS THERE

_____

_____

_____

_____

_____

_____

THE EXPERIENCE

_____
_____
_____
_____
_____
_____
_____
_____
_____
_____
_____

☆ ☆ ☆ ☆ ☆

address book

Name	Email	Cell

address book

Name	Email	Cell

address book

Name	Email	Cell

61131941R00064